Finding a Kidney

Finding a Kidney

And Getting the Most
Out of Your Transplant

Garet Hil

To order additional copies of this book, contact:
Xlibris Corporation
1-888-795-4274
www.Xlibris.com
Orders@Xlibris.com
94351

CONTENTS

Forward

I AM PLEASED AND excited that Garet Hil has created a comprehensive guide for people facing end stage renal disease (ESRD) who are in need of a kidney transplant. Garet has spent the majority of his time over the last three years dedicating himself to improving the process of living donor paired exchange. This passion is driven by personal experience (read about it in the "Our Story" chapter). That personal experience and drive led to the creation of the National Kidney Registry and this book. *Finding a Kidney* is an important resource for those who wish to put themselves in the position to receive the best possible outcome from the kidney transplant experience.

A few words about my own transplant experience may interest the readers of *Finding a Kidney*. I was in need of a kidney for the first time in 1995. I was a 26 year old with not a care in the world until I heard the words "You have kidney failure and you need to get to a hospital now." It's been 15 years since that statement, along with "We need to put you on dialysis A.S.A.P" and "A kidney transplant is your best option," was first uttered. If you're reading this book, you have probably heard these words or something just like them. SCARY!

I have had two living donor kidney transplants. The first came in 1996 from my dad and the second in 2010 from my wife. My dad was a direct donor. My wife was not a match. SCARY again! My transplant center then entered us in to the National Kidney Registry. I was transplanted 120 days after being entered. Both my wife and dad are doing well.

I tell you this story for two reasons:

1) I couldn't ask them to donate a kidney to me. I wouldn't know how. Who am I to ask someone to donate a kidney? They both *offered* to donate.

2) I didn't know that the National Kidney Registry even existed until five months post transplant. My perception was that I was being entered in to my transplant center's swap program. I am one of the lucky ones (you will understand how lucky after you read this book) and am grateful every minute of every day. But the point of my story is this: don't rely on luck. Educate yourself.

Garet Hil clearly outlines the process that he has created from years of personal experience, tireless research and alignment with some of the most forward thinking physicians in the transplant community. I'm sure that some readers will have creative ideas to find a donor and I encourage that. This book is an educated guideline to be used in conjunction with your own ideas. *Finding a Kidney* is an immensely useful step-by-step guide for people who wish to help themselves.

Finally, this book reflects the intelligence and passion of the author, whose drive and enthusiasm has been a gift not only to his daughter but to all people in need of a kidney transplant.

Gary LeBlanc

Introduction

WHEN WE WERE faced with the challenge of finding a donor for our 10-year-old daughter, we entered the complex and confusing world that confronts most people in need of a kidney. I wish there were a book like this back then to translate into layman's terms all of the things we needed to know and eventually learned the hard way. This book attempts to fill the void and explain in simple terms how to find a kidney and get the most out of your transplant.

Our Story

WHEN MY YOUNGEST daughter was 10 years old, her kidneys failed. When we learned that she would never recover her kidney function, it was clear that a living donor kidney transplant would give her the best outcome. My wife, who knew her own blood type— she was a "B"— and was not a compatible donor. Our daughter was an "A" blood type and "B" blood types are not compatible with "A"s. I did not know my blood type so I raced home to check my old military records to find my blood type and see if I was compatible. I was overcome with relief when I discovered that we were both "A" blood types and I would be able to donate.

I immediately went to my doctor to see if I was medically qualified to donate. Everything looked good, but my blood pressure was higher than normal so I ramped up my workout schedule to two to four hours a day, seven days a week. When my doctor measured my blood pressure after a few weeks, it had increased! This was baffling and terrifying because high blood pressure could rule me out as a donor. He then sent me home with a 24-hour blood pressure monitor so we could see where my blood pressure was when I was out of his office. That did the trick. I had "white coat syndrome." I knew that if my blood pressure was high, it would keep me from donating and there was nothing more important than being able to donate my kidney to my little girl.

To be safe, I was tested along with three of her uncles. All four of us passed the tests and three of us were three-antigen matches—pretty good matches and typical of the match between parents and their kids. Now we were even more secure. Not only could I donate, but we had a good bench in case something went wrong and I could not donate to my daughter.

The surgery was scheduled for a Thursday in the middle of May. That Monday, we received a call from the transplant center letting us know there was a problem and we needed to return to the center to do another crossmatch test. We went in early the next morning, took the additional crossmatch test, and waited. Late Tuesday afternoon, 36 hours prior to surgery, we received another call. I had failed the crossmatch test again. Surgery was canceled. I could not donate because my daughter would reject my kidney. She had developed a potent antibody against my B60 antigen. I had become antibody incompatible.

In the weeks that followed, all of the uncles that were initially tested failed subsequent crossmatch tests. At the same time an anonymous Good Samaritan donor stepped forward—she was also a three-antigen match with my daughter. After another trip to the hospital and another crossmatch test, we learned that the anonymous donor had also failed the crossmatch test. We had gone from five blood compatible donors to none in just a few weeks.

This was a dark time. In response to this crisis, my wife and I worked around the clock to recruit and test additional donors. We also attempted to enter ourselves in every kidney exchange program in the United States. None of these paired exchange programs were able to find a match for our daughter. Several programs did not even return my many phone calls and some of them wanted to force our daughter to switch to far away hospitals to enter their exchange program. This is when we realized the incredible undeveloped potential of paired exchange and decided to start a national kidney registry.

In the end, after screening 15 potential direct donors, we found one who was compatible and could donate. It was my daughter's 23-year-old cousin. He cleared all the hurdles, was an excellent match, and donated his kidney in July of 2007. Both my daughter and my brave and generous nephew are doing well.

So You Need a New Kidney

DON'T FREAK OUT—you are not alone. Over 100,000 people in the United States are walking around with a transplanted kidney in them and are leading full, productive lives. It is not a new or novel procedure and the outcomes are excellent if you take good care of your transplanted kidney.

If you are reading this book, it's likely that you have an interest in finding a kidney for yourself or someone you love. I wrote this book to help you improve your chances of finding that kidney and to increase the odds that your transplanted kidney will last as long as possible.

The first decision you must make is a multi-layered one. Do you want a transplant? And, if you do want a transplant, do you want a living donor transplant or a deceased donor transplant? Below is a diagram of this simple decision tree.

Figure 1 – Kidney Failure Options

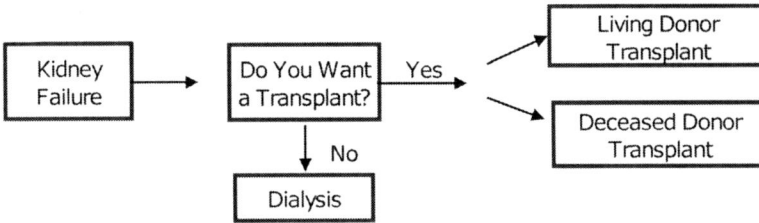

```
┌──────────┐      ┌──────────────┐  Yes      ┌──────────────────┐
│ Kidney   │─────▶│ Do You Want  │──────────▶│ Living Donor     │
│ Failure  │      │ a Transplant?│           │ Transplant       │
└──────────┘      └──────────────┘           └──────────────────┘
                         │                   ┌──────────────────┐
                         │ No                │ Deceased Donor   │
                         ▼                   │ Transplant       │
                   ┌──────────┐              └──────────────────┘
                   │ Dialysis │
                   └──────────┘
```

I will spend no time reviewing the pros and cons of dialysis versus a transplant. If you have picked up this book you have most likely already made the decision to go for a transplant. In most cases a transplant provides a better quality of life and longer life expectancy, but I have met people who have made the choice to stay on dialysis and are leading full, healthy lives. I remember meeting a 70-year old man, when my daughter was still on dialysis, who had been on dialysis for almost a decade and enjoyed his naps while he was dialyzing at home. This guy swam five days a week and was the picture of health. He was the exception, but proved to me that it is possible to live well on dialysis.

The next logical question, then, is "should I go for a deceased donor transplant or living donor transplant?" These are very different processes with different outcomes. Generally, if you have a living donor, you will have a better outcome. Even if your living donor is incompatible, you can do a swap and get a well matched living donor kidney transplant.

By far, a living donor transplant lasts much longer than a deceased donor transplant. Below is a chart that shows the graft half-life of living donor kidney transplants and deceased donor kidney transplants.

Figure 2 – How Long Transplanted Kidneys Typically Last

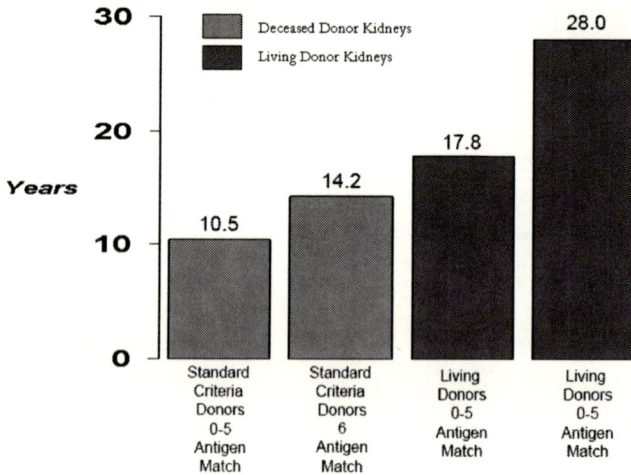

Source: Clinical Transplants 2005

In addition to the difference in how long the kidneys last, living donor transplants have the following advantages over deceased donor transplants:

- There is no inherent wait time in getting a living donor kidney transplant, whereas wait time for deceased donor kidneys runs between one and 15 years depending mostly on the transplant center you choose and the geographic location of that transplant center.

- There is a significantly higher probability that a living donor kidney will be functioning after 1, 3, 5, 10 and 20 years.

- Living donor surgery can be scheduled in advance as opposed to deceased donor surgery that can happen at any time, requiring you to be "on call" for years.

If living donor transplants are so much better than deceased donor transplants, why are there more deceased donor transplants in the U.S. than living donor transplants? The answer is simple. The recipient cannot find a donor. Based on my conversations with hundreds of recipients and donors, I believe that many have just not asked the right person the right question (we cover this in more detail in the "Your Donor Campaign" chapter).

As with dialysis, there are many people who have received deceased donor kidneys and are leading healthy and full lives. But the sad reality is that the demand for deceased donor kidneys continues to outstrip the supply, and average wait time for deceased donor kidneys has been getting longer every year. So, if you can, I encourage you to pursue a living donor transplant while still registering on the deceased donor list as a fallback plan so that you accrue "wait time" points in the deceased donor system while you search for a living donor.

Setting Yourself Up To Win

LIKE ANY MAJOR change in your life, you need to make finding a kidney a priority, and you need to set yourself up to win. The first step toward this goal involves finding a patient-focused transplant center (and several back-up centers) and immediately getting in there for tests that will determine if you are "qualified" for a transplant. The definition of "qualified" differs by transplant center so do not be discouraged if a center tells you that you are not qualified (e.g. you are too fat, you don't have the right insurance, etc.). There are over 250 transplant centers in the United States—many to choose from.

While you are working toward medical clearance at your transplant center, you need to launch your donor campaign. During this process you will experience up days and down days, but stay focused on finding a kidney and make sure that your life is organized to achieve this goal.

If you have antibodies (i.e. you are sensitized) it will be harder to find a compatible donor. Antibodies are created from sensitization events which include transplants, blood transfusions, and pregnancies. Avoid sensitization events, if possible, and redo your blood test after any sensitization event so that you and your transplant center know your

Panel Reactive Antibodies (PRA) score and exactly which antibodies you have. You generally cannot receive a kidney from someone who has an antigen that is the same as one of your antibodies. This will cause a crossmatch failure.

One common pitfall that my wife and I experienced, which we see often among the people we work with, is the "I have a donor" syndrome. You DO NOT have a donor until the day of the surgery. There are many reasons a donor can fall out of the process—sometimes at the last minute. I learned 36 hours prior to surgery that I could not donate to my daughter because of an unexpected crossmatch failure. We have seen donors back out of the process or become ill just days before surgery. We have even seen donors discover they are pregnant before surgery, ruling them out. We have seen recipients announce that they have a donor and eliminate other donors who have stepped forward, only to find out later that their "donor" has a horse-shoe kidney and is ruled out. So remember, anything can happen. You don't have a donor until the day of surgery.

We have also seen many recipients get called in numerous times, often in the middle of the night, for deceased donor transplants, only to be sent home after someone else got the kidney. Many centers bring in two to four recipients for every deceased donor kidney to ensure the kidney can be used if someone doesn't show up or if the recipient fails the crossmatch. Adopt a mindset of having "many horses in the race." This way, if one transplant opportunity falls through, you always have a backup.

If you have not done so already, you should sign up for Medicare Part A as soon as possible. Most people who have paid taxes and have end stage renal disease (i.e. kidney failure) are covered by Medicare Part A. If you have private insurance, that is even better because private insurance pays the hospitals more money for the transplant services than Medicare. There will likely be a social worker at your dialysis center or a financial advisor at your transplant center who will help you complete the applications and explain the details of how the transplant and immunosuppressive drugs are covered. This is what they get paid for, so don't hesitate to ask them any questions you may have.

Finally, set yourself up to win by staying healthy and focusing on a positive outcome. Put on hold the other things in your life that may be generating stress. Make sure you are getting enough sleep, eating right, exercising and following you doctor's instructions. Consider what an athlete does before competing in the Olympics. Your outcome is no less important than winning a gold medal.

Living Donor Kidney Transplants

NOW IT IS time to learn about living donor kidney transplants and some of the medical lingo. Once you find someone who is willing to become a living donor, he or she will be tested by your transplant center and will fall into one of the following categories:

- Medically unqualified to donate
- Medically qualified, but incompatible
- Medically qualified & compatible

It is estimated that 40%—60% of the donors interviewed by transplant centers are medically unqualified to donate. The most common disqualifications are high blood pressure, diabetes and obesity. Often donors are categorized as medically unqualified when the donors indicate to the transplant center that they are not willing to go through with the surgery. This allows the donors to gracefully exit the donor evaluation process.

Approximately 50% of the donors that are medically qualified will be incompatible with the recipient. When we were seeking a compatible donor for our daughter, we screened 15 potential donors and only two were ultimately compatible with our daughter. There are two primary reasons that a donor is incompatible: blood type incompatibility and antibody incompatibility. Below is a table that shows the compatible and incompatible blood type combinations.

Figure 3 – Blood Type Compatibilities

		O	A	B	AB
Recipient Blood Type	O	Compatible	Incompatible	Incompatible	Incompatible
	A	Compatible	Compatible	Incompatible	Incompatible
	B	Compatible	Incompatible	Compatible	Incompatible
	AB	Compatible	Compatible	Compatible	Compatible

As you can see, "O" blood types are universal donors and can give a kidney to anyone. "AB" blood types are universal recipients and can get a kidney from any blood group. It is hardest to find a compatible donor if you are an "O" blood type and easiest if you are an "AB" blood type.

Antibody incompatibility is the second type of incompatibility. The only recipients that fail crossmatches (i.e. antibody incompatible) are those who have undergone a sensitization event. There are three primary types of sensitization events:

- Prior Transplants
- Blood Transfusions
- Pregnancy

GARET HIL

We have come across a few situations where tattoos and vaccines seem to have created antibodies in a recipient but this is rare and there does not seem to be any research on this.

I failed the crossmatch with my daughter because she received blood transfusions when her kidneys failed, so if you think you will need a kidney transplant someday, AVOID BLOOD TRANSFUSIONS. Mothers often have antibodies (are sensitized) against their children. This is why fathers who receive kidneys from their children have significantly better outcomes than mothers who receive kidneys from their children. Mothers that have children who want to donate to them should ALWAYS consider paired exchange so they can create an opportunity to get a better matched donor.

If you have had a prior transplant, and it was a six-antigen match, you will not create antibodies since the human body generally does not create antibodies against its own antigens (unless the patient has an auto immune disease). This is one of the reasons it is important to get a well matched kidney, if possible, especially for young people who may need another transplant in their lifetime. The better the match, the fewer antibodies are created and the easier it is to get a second or third transplant in the future.

What do you do if you have an incompatible donor? Ten years ago there was little you *could* do, but today you have several options. The first is to "swap" your incompatible donor to get a donor who is compatible. This is done through a "paired exchange." The first recorded paired exchange in the United States occurred in 2000. Since then, over a thousand transplants have been facilitated through paired exchanges. New innovations in paired exchanges are not only facilitating more transplants for incompatible donor/recipient pairs but are improving the donor match for compatible pairs (more on this in the "Paired Exchange" chapter).

If you have an incompatible donor, your second option is to undergo desensitization. Although better than dialysis, this has been demonstrated to have poor long term outcomes (i.e. five plus years) and should be considered only as a last resort. If your transplant center is selling you on their desensitization program but does not have a productive paired exchange program, you should find another center.

Finally, many centers are combining paired exchange with desensitization for those patients that are very highly sensitized. This is the most powerful approach for getting really hard-to-match patients transplanted. If you have a high PRA (greater than 80%) you should seek out a center that combines paired exchange with desensitization. Just last year we were able to find a six-antigen match (perfect) for a patient that had a 99.9% PRA. This does not happen often, but in this case the recipient beat one-in-a-thousand odds of finding a compatible donor, and did not require any desensitization.

The last donor category is someone who is medically qualified and compatible. These potential donors are your best transplant opportunity, but as I must remind you, there is no such thing as a sure thing. You always want to have backups in case your primary donor falls through. In many cases, you can improve the donor match by participating in a paired exchange even when you have a compatible donor.

For example, let's say that you, as an unsensitized "A" blood type, need a kidney and your mother wants to donate. She is an "O" blood type. In this scenario, it is possible that you can find a better match in a paired exchange. Even though your mother is biologically related and will likely be a three-antigen match, you may be able to find a younger and/or larger donor with the same or better antigen match. We just found such a match as this book was going to press, proving that even parent/child matches can be improved upon.

The easiest donor/recipient matches to improve upon through swaps are unsensitized (i.e. no antibodies) patients with "AB", "A" and "B" blood types that have "O" donors. In fact, in these cases it is highly likely that the match can be improved, resulting in a kidney transplant that lasts longer.

A paired exchange transplant can take three to 12 weeks to set up after match offers have been accepted by all participants. If you have a compatible donor and your donor is giving to you directly, your transplant center should be able to complete your surgery within six weeks. If they cannot fit you into their schedule within six weeks, you may want to consider going to another transplant center. Remember, speed matters for the best outcome.

Deceased Donor Kidney Transplants

I F YOU HAVE read the prior chapter, you are now familiar with living donor transplants. Here you will learn the basics about deceased donor transplants. Deceased donor kidneys are removed from people who have died and who consented to donate their organs upon death to help others. Generally, deceased donor kidneys are removed from the donor and transplanted into a recipient 10 to 30 hours after removal.

As I have said earlier in this book, if you need a kidney, I believe you should have several horses in the race. I recommend that you get yourself on the deceased donor list as fast as possible so you can start accumulating wait time points regardless of whether or not you have potential living donors. If you are confident that you will get a living donor kidney, you can always turn down a deceased donor kidney offer while you continue to pursue your living donor transplant. You can also list yourself in the deceased donor system so that you will only get called if you get offered a six-antigen-matched kidney from standard criteria donors.

If your primary focus is to get a deceased donor transplant, there are several things you should know that will improve your odds of getting a deceased donor kidney.

First, wait time for a deceased donor kidney varies widely by geographic region in the U.S. and by transplant center within each geographic region. If you have the time and resources, you can list at the centers that have shorter wait times but you will need to be in a position to get to that center quickly (in under six hours) if you get an offer for a deceased donor kidney. You can list at multiple centers in different regions but not multiple centers in the same region. For example, you can list at a New York center and also at a New Jersey center, but you cannot list at two New York centers. California is organized into two regions so you can list at one San Francisco center and one Los Angeles center, but you cannot list at two San Francisco centers. The longest wait times, by far, are in California, Texas and parts of the southeast where 10 plus years is common. However, there are many centers in the U.S. with wait time under three years.

Where do you find this information and what is the formula for expected wait time? Although it is very difficult to navigate, all of the wait list information can be found on the government's Web site at *http://optn.transplant.hrsa.gov/*. Here you can look up the median wait time by transplant center to get a very rough sense of the expected wait time. The problem with the way this site calculates median wait time is that it measures wait times using a rear view mirror approach— based on transplant candidates that were listed three to 10 years ago—so it may not be a good predictor of the wait times you can expect going forward.

The best measure we have found for determining the expected wait time looking forward is to divide the center's current wait list by the number of deceased donor kidney transplants that a center is completing annually and then cut that number in half to reflect the wait list attrition. For example, if a center has a wait list of 1,000 patients and they are doing 100 deceased donor transplants annually, that center will have an expected wait time of five years (1,000 reduced by half to 500 divided by 100 = 5 years). Using this simple formula, you will find that some centers have average wait times in excess of 15 years and others have expected wait times of less than three years.

Who gets the kidney? The allocation of deceased donor kidneys is managed by the United Network for Organ Sharing (UNOS) under contract with the government. The allocation process is very complex but, at its core, directs kidneys to people who have waited the longest. Priority is given to children, who generally get offered a kidney in less than two years. The points awarded to children don't disappear when they turn 18, so these patients can roll over their points, eliminating the "use it or lose it" stress related to turning 19. Also, although it rarely happens, it is important to note that living kidney donors are automatically given priority on the deceased donor wait list, allowing them to get deceased donor kidneys very quickly if they ever need one.

There are some practical considerations to keep in mind when you are waiting for a deceased donor kidney. First of all, make sure your transplant center can reach you 24/7. Many people lose the opportunity to get transplanted simply because they don't answer the phone. Also, you must make sure all of your medical records are updated at the transplant center so that you do not lose an offer because the center's paperwork is not current. Many centers literally have thousands of patients on their wait list, making it impossible for staff to follow you on an individual basis. You must be your own advocate.

Improving Your Odds

I N THIS CHAPTER we review all the ways that you can improve your odds of getting a great transplant outcome. But first we need to define what a "great outcome" is. A great outcome is a transplant that lasts a long time (20+ years) with minimal complications and negative side effects. We will use the measurement of "graft survival" to determine the impact of certain factors that will improve your odds for a great outcome. Graft survival is simply a measurement of the percentage of recipients that still have a functioning kidney at a given point in time (e.g. 10 years) after the transplant. For example a 95% graft survival rate after 10 years would indicate that 95 out of 100 recipients still have a functioning graft 10 years after transplantation. This would be a very good graft survival rate whereas a 40% graft survival rate after three years would be a bad graft survival rate.

The first thing someone facing kidney failure can do to improve the odds of a great outcome (if you can see kidney failure coming) is to get a pre-emptive transplant. This means that you receive a transplant before you ever go on dialysis. Because of the long wait times for deceased donor kidneys, a pre-emptive transplant is usually only available to recipients that have living donors. Not only does a pre-emptive transplant keep you off dialysis, but it increases the five year graft survival by about five percent. Pre-emptive transplants have only become mainstream since about 2005. In fact, there was a time, not so long ago, when Medicare and the insurance companies would not pay for a transplant unless the patient was already on dialysis.

The graft survival rate studies indicate that once you are on dialysis, the first six months of dialysis has no statistically significant negative effect on graft survival, but once the first six months passes, graft survival rates start to decline. Once you know you will need a kidney transplant, you need to move fast—TIME MATTERS. Since most deceased donor wait times are much greater than six months, this fast mover advantage is typically only available if you have a living donor.

If you are lucky enough to have more than one potential living donor, you can increase your odds by choosing a donor that is the best match for you. You can also improve your donor match by entering into a swap to get a better match (see the "Paired Exchange" chapter). Although there may be some differences in donor matches, it is a BAD strategy to hold out for a better donor if that means significantly delaying your transplant. The benefits of a living donor transplant versus staying on dialysis are so significant that they vastly outweigh the benefits of finding a slightly better matched donor. Time matters. The faster you can get your transplant, the better off you are.

There are four factors related to donor selection that appear to have the most impact on a successful transplant outcome. They are:

- Donor age
- Donor/recipient antigen match
- Relative size of the donor to the recipient
- Donor commitment

The age of the donor has an impact on graft survival rates. If you have two donors that are equal in all ways except one is 20 years younger than the other, then the younger donor kidney is likely to last longer. Also, the effects of donor age on graft survival do not become pronounced until the donor is 65 years old or older. In other words, there is little difference between a 25 and 35 year old donor but a big difference between a 60 and 70 year old donor.

Figure 4 – Living Donor Transplant Graft Survival Rate by Donor Age at 10 Years

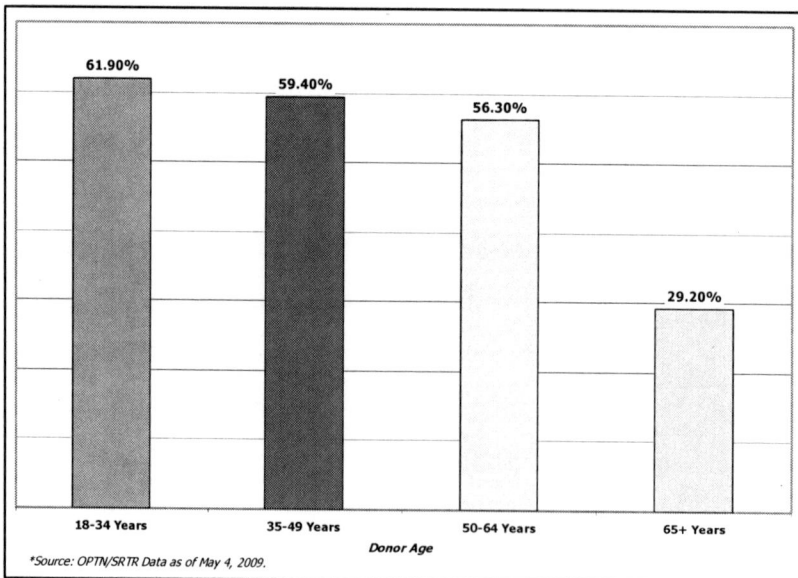

Donor Age: 18-34 Years: 61.90%, 35-49 Years: 59.40%, 50-64 Years: 56.30%, 65+ Years: 29.20%

*Source: OPTN/SRTR Data as of May 4, 2009.

Figure 5 – Deceased Donor Transplant Graft Survival Rate by Donor Age at 10 Years

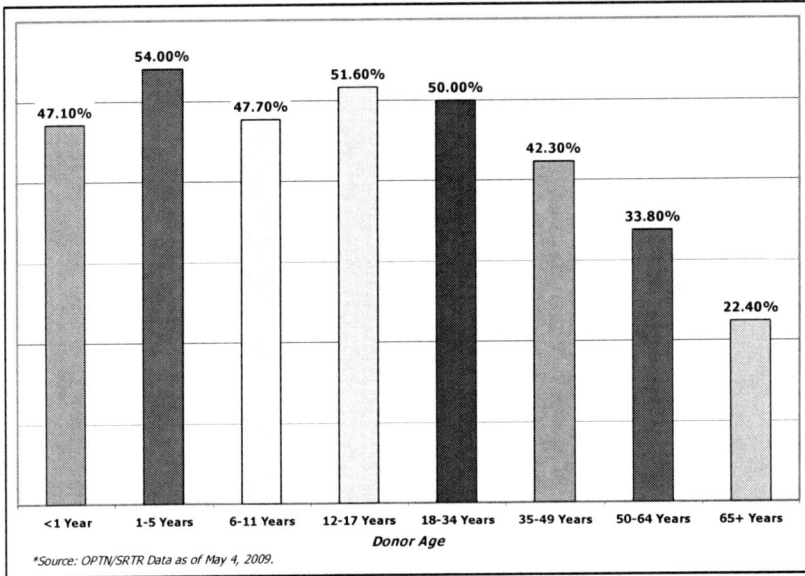

Bar chart showing graft survival rates by donor age:
- <1 Year: 47.10%
- 1-5 Years: 54.00%
- 6-11 Years: 47.70%
- 12-17 Years: 51.60%
- 18-34 Years: 50.00%
- 35-49 Years: 42.30%
- 50-64 Years: 33.80%
- 65+ Years: 22.40%

Donor Age

*Source: OPTN/SRTR Data as of May 4, 2009.

The antigen match between donors and recipients is another important factor impacting graft survival. The best match is a six-antigen match and is very rare, occurring between siblings 25% of the time and always between identical twins. Parents and siblings generally match on three antigens. The worst antigen match is zero and is fairly common between unrelated donors and recipients. To put this into perspective, a zero-antigen-matched living donor still has a much better graft survival rate than a six-antigen-matched deceased donor kidney, so even a zero-matched living donor will likely yield a great outcome.

Figure 6 – Living Donor Transplant
Graft Survival Rate by HLA Match at 10 Years

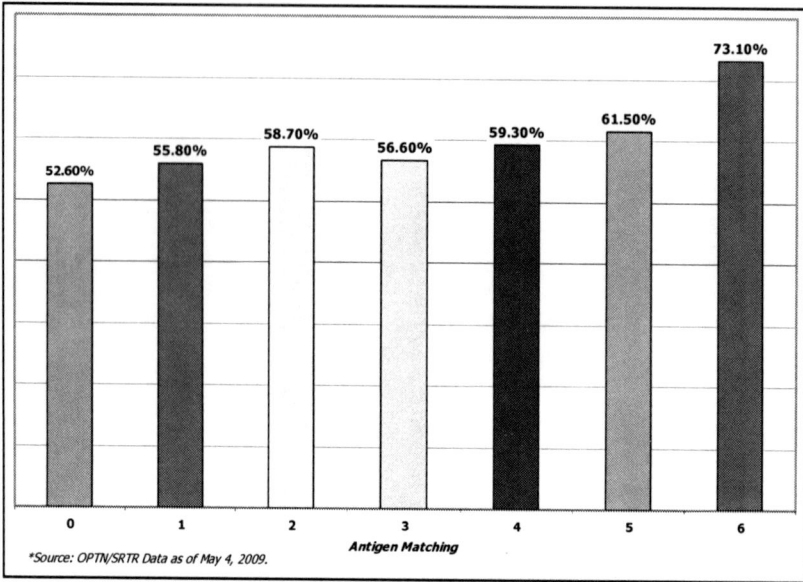

52.60% **55.80%** **58.70%** **56.60%** **59.30%** **61.50%** **73.10%**

0   1   2   3   4   5   6

Antigen Matching

Source: OPTN/SRTR Data as of May 4, 2009.

Figure 7 – Deceased Donor Transplant
Graft Survival Rate by HLA Match at 10 Years

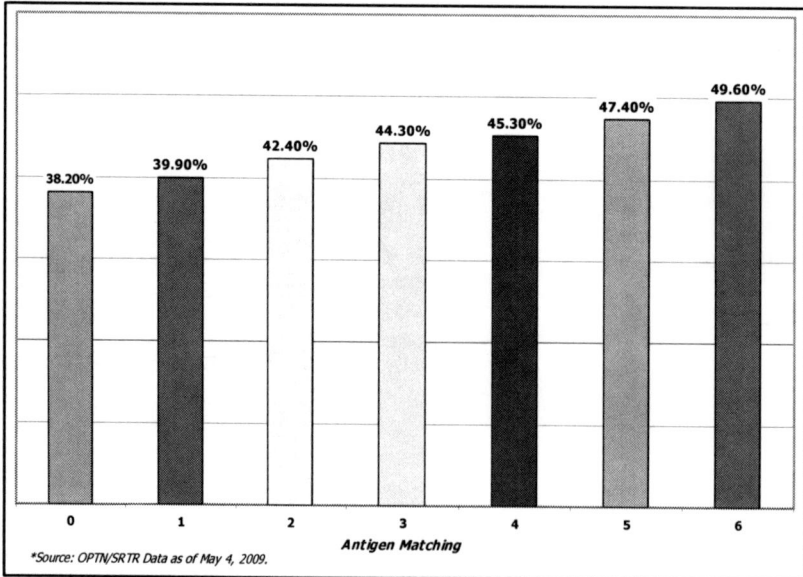

38.20% **39.90%** **42.40%** **44.30%** **45.30%** **47.40%** **49.60%**

0   1   2   3   4   5   6

Antigen Matching

Source: OPTN/SRTR Data as of May 4, 2009.

The relative size of the donor may also be important. Generally, the bigger the donor, the larger the kidney and the longer the kidney may last. This situation has not been researched thoroughly but sometimes transplant centers will recommend against transplanting a kidney from a small donor (e.g. 95 pound woman) into a large recipient (e.g. 250 pound man). More research is needed on this front but the following chart from research published in 2003 indicates that size does matter.

Figure 8 – Living Donor Transplant Graft Survival Rate by Donor/Recipient Size Ratio at 5 Years

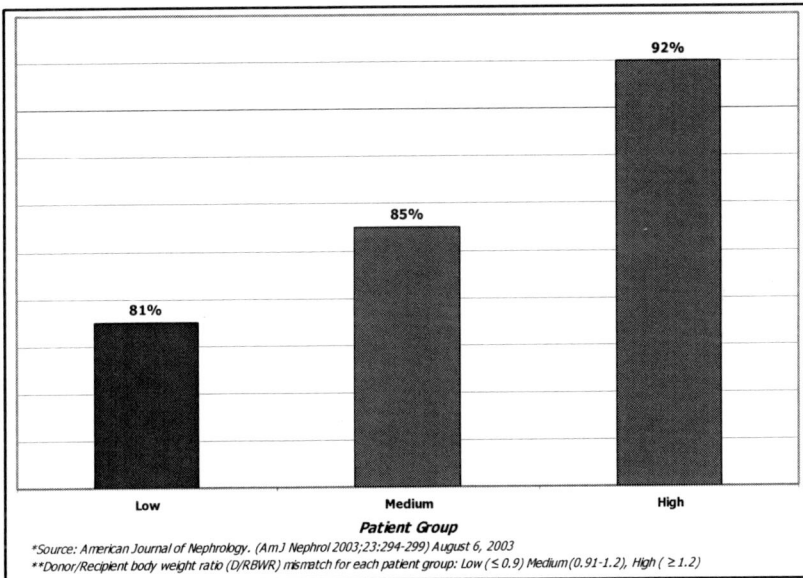

*Source: American Journal of Nephrology. (Am J Nephrol 2003;23:294-299) August 6, 2003
**Donor/Recipient body weight ratio (D/RBWR) mismatch for each patient group: Low (≤ 0.9) Medium (0.91-1.2), High (≥ 1.2)

When evaluating living donors, you must also consider the commitment of the donor. I have seen many cases in which a donor says that he wants to donate but then backs out of the process as the surgery date nears. You may have a donor who is a great match, but if he is unlikely to actually go through with the donation then you are better off focusing your efforts on other donors. Remember, time matters.

Finally, stay healthy and maintain a positive mental attitude. If you are overweight, take the opportunity now to lose the extra weight. Make sure you eat right, exercise, and get enough sleep. If you have other health problems, follow your doctor's instructions. Think of the transplant as an athletic event for which you must prepare in advance for a great performance. Much of the outcome is under your control, so stay focused and you will achieve a great outcome.

Running an Effective Donor Campaign

WHAT IS AN effective donor campaign and how do you manage one? First, you must build a team for the donor search and transplant process. Ideally this team should include an administrator, a caregiver, and one or more donor recruiters. In many cases, one person may have more than one role on this team. For example, a spouse may be the administrator and the caregiver while the parents are the recruiters. It is best if the recipient focuses on his/her mental and physical health prior to transplant and does not try to take on these roles unless there is no one to fill them. The administrator will manage all the insurance, medical records, and other paperwork, which must be well organized. The caregiver will oversee the recipient's medical needs. The recruiter(s) will focus on finding donors for either direct donation or paired donation. For our daughter's situation, I was the administrator, my wife was the caregiver and we both shared the recruiter role.

Choose your recruiters thoughtfully. The best recruiters will generally be people close to the recipient who cannot donate because they have already donated a kidney or they cannot donate for health reasons (e.g. age). Have your recruiters start working immediately. Have cards printed to give to potential donors. The cards should have the phone number of the transplant center, the name of the transplant center and coordinator; and the name of the patient. Keep an updated list of potential donors and review the list weekly with the transplant center. You and your recruiter have limited time, so focus on the potential donors who are healthy, committed, and may be willing to enter into a paired exchange.

You cannot "sell" people into donation—taking this approach will not be effective. Most people who donate made the decision long ago or were already pre-disposed to donate. It is generally best not to initially ask if someone will donate—people need time to do the research and understand what it means to donate. Give potential donors a Web site as a starting point for this research. A good Web site for this research is *www.transplantliving.org.* Instead of initially asking if someone will donate, ask the potential donor if they would consider being tested to determine if they can donate. Some people say they will consider being tested but never follow through—expect this. This is an effective screen to determine whether someone is serious about donating.

Do not convince yourself or tell anyone that you have a donor during the search process. Until the surgery actually takes place, you only have potential donors. There are many reasons that potential donors never become actual donors—medical and otherwise. It may turn out that even though you have 10 potential donors, none of them can donate. Do not stop recruiting even if you have several potential donors that have cleared the medical work-up process. Do not stop recruiting until your potential donor has passed the final crossmatch test that generally takes place one week from the surgery date.

If you are a recruiter, ask everyone you know if they would consider donating. Start with family (siblings have the best chance of being great matches) and friends and build from there. Whenever you ask people if they would consider donating, regardless of their willingness to donate, follow up by asking if they know of anyone who may be willing to donate.

Big hearted, brave people are the most likely to donate. If someone is, or was, in a courageous profession such as law enforcement, the military, or firefighting, they are more likely to consider donating. These people generally have many brave friends who may be willing to donate even though they do not know the recipient.

Ideally, every potential donor who is willing to donate directly would also be willing to donate through an exchange. However, this is not always the case. Sometimes a donor will be willing to donate directly but not through a paired exchange. You need to determine this at the appropriate time so that you will know if the donor can still help if they are found to be incompatible with the recipient.

Donors who are willing to enter into an exchange are powerful because they do not need to be blood compatible or antibody compatible with you. These donors are also powerful because they can expose the recipient to hundreds of other potential donors. The more donors you can be exposed to through an exchange, the greater the opportunity for an excellent match. When entering an exchange program, "O" donors are the most powerful of all when it comes to compatibility with patients who are hard to match because there is a shortage of "O" donors in all exchange programs.

Finally, many people are confused about what expenses the recipient can cover for the donor. The transplant industry is very sensitive to the topic of donor compensation because it is illegal in the United States. Sometimes transplant centers unknowingly discourage reimbursement of donor costs because of institutional paranoia linked to the illegality of compensating donors. Reimbursing donor expenses is a very different issue than donor compensation and is completely legal, and in some cases necessary.

Donors will have many costs directly related to their donation. Because of the altruistic nature of living donation, and the generous nature of donors, many donors refuse to be reimbursed for donation-related expenses. However, many donors do not have the financial resources to absorb the costs incurred through donation and must be reimbursed in order to donate.

The most common donation-related expenses are lost wages during the donation and recovery period, travel, lodging, and costs related to post transplant medical follow-ups. If you have the resources to cover or defray your donor's expenses, let your potential donors know. Many times a few thousand dollars in lost wages and travel costs will deter a potential donor from offering to donate.

Choosing Your Transplant Center

T HE MEDICAL TEAM you select for your transplant can have a significant impact on your transplant outcome. Your medical team should consist of a transplant nephrologist, a surgeon, and a transplant nurse/coordinator. This medical team will usually work at, or be related to, the transplant center you choose—so choose wisely. There are over 250 transplant centers in the United States from which to make your selection. The key things to look for include:

- *Do they take your insurance?* Since 50% of transplant patients are covered by Medicare and all transplant centers take Medicare, this insurance question is only relevant to those that have private insurance.
- *Proximity*: You will be going back and forth to the center a lot (before and after the transplant) and you may need to get to your transplant team fast if you have complications. If you choose a center that is far from your home, you should consider renting a place near the center to live for one to three months following the transplant to ensure quick access to your team.
- *Non-Steroidal Immunosuppressants*: Many centers offer newer non-steroid therapies for immunosuppressants

after transplantation. The side effects of steroid based immuno-supression can be significant and adverse over the long term. This is an especially important consideration for children.

- *Successful Track Record*: This is generally measured by what is called "graft survival" and can be found at *www.ustransplant.org*. Keep in mind that sometimes top centers can end up with lower graft survival rates because they take on the most challenging cases.

- *Paired Exchange:* If you have a living donor that is incompatible or you want to enter a swap to get a more favorably matched donor, you will want to go to a transplant center that is good at paired exchange. For a list of NKR member centers and their paired exchange results, go to *www.kidneyregistry.org*.

- *Desensitization:* If you have a living donor and you are highly sensitized, your best opportunity will be to go to a center that is good at paired exchange AND desensitization.

- *Wait Times:* If you do not have a living donor and want to get transplanted quickly, the center's expected wait time will be an important selection criterion. Please see the "Deceased Donor Transplant" chapter for more information on understanding wait times by center.

After your surgery, you must absolutely take your medications as directed. Taking all the different medications after surgery can be a complex and challenging task. You may want to consider getting a pillbox with an alarm on it for assistance in taking your medications on time. If you are looking for a Web site that offers a variety of pillbox alarm systems, you can try *www.epill.com*. Just as getting a well-matched living donor is the most important controllable factor for a great transplant outcome, taking your medications accurately and on time after getting your new kidney is the most important post-transplant factor for sustaining that great outcome.

If you end up back in the hospital for post-operative complications, take your medications with you to the hospital. Never blindly trust anyone, including the hospital staff, to give you your medications. They sometimes make mistakes. You may need to rush back to the hospital and check into the emergency room if you have complications, so keep a bag packed and by the door. Be prepared to leave at any moment. If the results from your routine blood tests come back with abnormalities, you will need to get to the emergency room quickly. If you need to return to the hospital because of complications, ask your surgeon or nephrologist to meet you in the emergency room. This will save you time and allow you to avoid potential mistakes made by other medical professionals who are not familiar with your situation.

Paired Exchange

THERE ARE THREE things you need to know about getting a kidney transplant through a paired exchange.

1) Who are the best candidates for paired exchange?
2) What donor characteristics matter the most?
3) Why does the transplant center you choose really matter?

Most people think that paired exchange is only for ESRD patients that have incompatible donors. This is no longer the case. Patients with poorly compatible donors and patients with compatible donors are also entering swaps to find better matched donors so their transplanted kidney will last longer. An example of a poorly matched donor may be someone who is more than 20 years older than the recipient or a recipient that has low level antibodies against the donor, as is often the case when a child wants to donate to their mother.

Even when a donor is completely compatible with the recipient, sometimes the recipient can improve the match by entering a swap. This strategy is most successful when an unsensitized (i.e. 0 PRA) "A", "B" or "AB" recipient has a blood type "O" donor. This is a very powerful combination in a swap and can improve the match, while facilitating up to a dozen additional transplants for those patients with incompatible donors.

Some patients have more than one incompatible donor. My daughter had 13 incompatible donors, including myself (antibody incompatible) and my wife (blood incompatible). If you have more than one incompatible donor willing to enter a swap, your most powerful donors will be young (i.e. less than 50 years old) "O" blood type donors. "B" is the next most powerful donor blood type, followed by "A" and "AB" blood types. "O" donors are more than 10 times more powerful than the other blood types, so if you are lucky enough to have several incompatible donors, try to get your "O" donors worked up and entered into the paired exchange system first. Other donor characteristics that impact the chance of finding a match in paired exchange include donor age, with donors less than 50 years old being the more powerful donors. Sometimes donor size matters (the bigger the better) but this is the least important characteristic. By far, the most important characteristic that can improve the probability of finding a match in a swap is being paired with a blood type "O" donor.

Many transplant centers claim they provide paired exchange services, but there are huge differences in paired exchange performance between centers. You want to ask the center three simple questions:

1) How many active pairs does the center have in its pool of incompatible pairs?
2) How many exchange transplants has the center completed in the last 12 months?

3) What percent of the center's incompatible pool have been transplanted since the program started?

Divide #1 by #2 and you will get a rough estimate of the average wait time for a center to get you transplanted in a swap. For example, if the center has a pool of 30 pairs and they have gotten 15 pairs transplanted in the past 12 months, the average wait time is two years (30 divided by 15). The best centers will have average wait times of less than a year. As a point of reference, the average wait time for all of the National Kidney Registry member centers is 11 months, with easy-to-match pairs going to transplant in under three months. The industry average wait time in paired exchange is approximately five years, so there are big differences between centers. The National Kidney Registry member centers have transplanted roughly 60% *www.kidneyregistry.org* of their incompatible pairs since the program started three years ago, so you can use that as a benchmark when evaluating centers relative to question #3.

In conclusion, paired exchange can not only help those people with incompatible donors, but is now helping people with compatible donors get better matches that will allow the transplanted kidneys to last longer. If you have multiple donors, they are not all equal. Try to have your most powerful donors worked up first. Finally, the transplant center you choose can make the difference between getting transplanted quickly through paired exchange or remaining on dialysis. Choose your transplant center wisely.

Summary

I F YOU ARE facing kidney failure and are interested in the miracle of a kidney transplant, you are not alone and there are many things that are under your control that will help you achieve a great transplant outcome. I sincerely hope this book has helped you in your transplant journey and encourage you to give us feedback on how we can make the next edition of this book even more useful. Please email your suggestions and stories to *administration@kidneyregistry.org*.

9 781456 868154